CURRICULUM GUIDE
to accompany **Mosby's**

Pharmacy
Technician

PRINCIPLES & PRACTICE

CURRICULUM GUIDE
to accompany **Mosby's**

Pharmacy Technician

PRINCIPLES & PRACTICE

TERESA HOPPER, BS, CPhT

Pharmacy Technician Consultant
Heald College
San Francisco, California

Prepared by

KATHY MOSCOU, BS, RPh, MPh Candidate

Pharmacy Technician Program Director
North Seattle Community College
Seattle, Washington

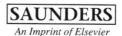

SAUNDERS
An Imprint of Elsevier

SAUNDERS
An Imprint of Elsevier

11830 Westline Industrial Drive
St. Louis, Missouri 63146

NOTICE

Pharmacology is an ever-changing field. Standard safety precautions must be followed, but as
new research and clinical experience broaden our knowledge, changes in treatment and drug
therapy may become necessary or appropriate. Readers are advised to check the most current
product information provided by the manufacturer of each drug to be administered to verify
the recommended dose, the method and duration of administration, and contraindications. It
is the responsibility of the licensed prescriber, relying on experience and knowledge of the
patient, to determine dosages and the best treatment for each individual patient. Neither the
publisher nor the author assumes any liability for any injury and/or damage to persons or
property arising from this publication.

International Standard Book Number 1-4160-0011-9

Executive Editor: Adrianne H. Cochran
Developmental Editor: Christine Ambrose
Publishing Services Manager: Melissa Lastarria
Senior Project Manager: Joy Moore
Designer: Amy Buxton

Printed in United States of America

Last digit is the print number: 9   8   7   6   5   4   3   2

Contents

Overview

The practice of pharmacy faces many challenges today. Pharmacy practice in the twenty-first century will undoubtedly require pharmacists to provide more cognitive services and drug utilization review (DUR) to an increasingly mobile population. Medications and services will most likely continue to be paid for by third-party insurance carriers if the current trend continues. According to the National Association of Chain Drug Stores (NACDS) estimates, the number of prescriptions will increase from 2.8 billion per year to 4 billion by the year 2005. In fact, the number of prescriptions will increase by 36%, but the number of pharmacists will increase by only 4.5%. The number of pharmacists is not projected to keep up with the demand. How can pharmaceutical care be provided, public health needs be met, and patient safety assured in the face of these challenges? Furthermore, how do we ensure that both present and future needs of the profession are addressed?

Pharmacists have relied on pharmacy technicians to perform duties since the mid-1940s.* Although pharmacy technicians are widely used, technicians receive varying levels of training before being hired. Currently, pharmacy technicians receive training in community and junior colleges, universities, vocational-technical schools, and on-the-job training programs. The length and scope of training vary significantly among programs. Indeed length of existing programs ranges between 540 hours and 2145 hours; the average length is approximately 970 hours.

Comprehensive training is crucial to the development of good pharmacy technicians. Many arguments can substantiate the call for comprehensive standardized training. Well-educated pharmacy technicians perform their job more effectively. Comprehensive standardized training for pharmacy technicians will enable them to perform more efficiently, skillfully, and accurately. Pharmacy technicians spend less time searching for drugs when they have good brand/generic name recognition, and pharmacists are interrupted less when technicians have been educated in appropriate warning label selection. Pharmacy technicians educated in pharmacology have the skills to identify the drug requested for refill when the patient can't remember the drug name. It is relatively common for patients to request a refill for their "water pill." A pharmacy technician who has received comprehensive training would be able to select the diuretic listed in the patient profile and confirm that it is the medication desired by the patient. Well-trained pharmacy technicians are able to effectively assist pharmacists in providing quality patient care because they have an understanding of drug interactions, therapeutic duplication, and excessive dose alerts screened by the computer. Moreover, these technicians recognize the importance of notifying the supervising pharmacist. Well-educated pharmacy technicians are more qualified to participate in Tech-Check-Tech, where pharmacy technicians check unit dose cart fill performed by another pharmacy technician, pharmacist final check is not required. This is permitted in some states concurrent with training and verification of accuracy. Well-educated pharmacy technicians recognize the importance of aseptic technique and make fewer mistakes preparing intravenous solutions. They are able to assist the pharmacist with recognition of dosage calculation errors and drug incompatibility errors.

Expanding the role of the pharmacy technician, thus enabling the pharmacist to play a greater role in providing patient care, may be the answer to the nation's problems of a growing volume of prescriptions, an aging population, and shortages of pharmacists and pharmacy technicians. This

---

*Mott D, Vanderpool W, Smeenk D: Ohio institutional pharmacy technicians' demographics and attitudes toward national voluntary pharmacy technician certification: an exploratory analysis, *J Pharm Technol* 15:18, 1999.

1

is why the National Community Pharmacists Association (NCPA) supports the use of pharmacy technicians in community pharmacies to enhance the pharmacist's role in providing quality pharmaceutical care. NCPA believes that proper training is critical to the health and safety of patients. The expansion of the role of pharmacy technicians, however, must be in tandem with standardized training and the institution of a national examination to determine competency.

Some would argue that on-the-job training must remain as a primary method of educating pharmacy technicians because no other opportunity for education exists in rural settings. The number of formal academic programs, however, has been rapidly expanding. According to the White Paper on Pharmacy Technicians: 2002, the number of academic programs in 2002 was approximately 247 schools in 42 states. This number continues to grow. Pharmacy Technician Educator Council (PTEC), a national organization composed of pharmacists, pharmacy technicians, and other credentialed pharmacy technician educators, chose college/vocational training over on-the-job training by more than three to one. PTEC recommends that (1) college/vocational educational programs should replace on-the-job training programs, (2) within 10 years, all technician training programs evolve into 2-year associate degree programs, and (3) hands-on training be continued as a necessary component of all training programs. Comprehensive education requires didactic and experiential components. Experiential learning should be acquired in both classroom-laboratory and on-the-job settings. Pharmacy technicians must learn the skills required for employment in ambulatory care and institutional practice settings and this training should be comprehensive, not job site specific.

Competency-Based Instruction

Because the goal of pharmacy technician education is to ensure mastery of skills needed to practice competently, training programs should be designed that use competency-based instruction. Clear training goals must be established and effective teaching methods used. Knowledge of the scope of practice of pharmacy technicians is essential to the development of instructional objectives.

Competency-based curriculum models are designed to create opportunities for skills attainment and to provide repetition to ensure mastery. Problem-based learning is essential to competency-based curriculum development. Curriculum developers should ask the following questions:

- What educational purposes are sought?
- What experiences can be provided to attain these purposes?
- How can training experiences be organized to ensure mastery?
- Does training provide learners the opportunity to apply knowledge to new situations, thus demonstrating critical thinking skills?
- How can skill mastery be evaluated?
- Do skills assessment methods require students to demonstrate mastery in ways that are observable to learners and the instructor?

Characteristics of Competency-Based Education

Competency-based educational models create opportunities for skills attainment and provide repetition to ensure mastery. Problem-based learning is essential to competency-based curriculum development. Effective and successful pharmacy technician programs have:

- Program learning goals that are defined
- Learning objectives with measurable standards
- Planned learning activities
- Teaching strategies for problem-based learning
- A learner-teacher partnership that redefines the role of instructor from "leader" to "facilitator"

Competency-Based Lessons

After a program has been developed that provides pharmacy technician students an opportunity to learn and practice skills needed to perform effectively in all pharmaceutical care settings, attention must given to designing lessons that ensure mastery of skills. Lessons should be designed that enable learners to understand why knowledge of skill is essential, how the skill is applied in the pharmacy setting, performance expectations, and practice to ensure mastery. Competency-based lessons:

- Are built on actual pharmacy technician performance expectations
- Have learning objectives with measurable outcomes
- Permit repetition of performance-related activities
- Simulate actual work-related situations
- Enable learners to think critically, problem-solve, and develop solutions
- Teach learners to monitor and evaluate their own performance (search for and correct their mistakes)
- Facilitate active, rather than passive learning
- Encourage self-learning
- Create opportunities for students to work with and learn from each other (emphasize team building)
- Emphasize hands-on, practical application of material

Competency-Based Assessment Tools

Various methods are available to assess the effectiveness of individual lessons, courses, or the entire pharmacy technician program. Program assessment is covered in detail in the section entitled Program Assessment. Classroom assessment techniques (CAT) are useful tools to obtain immediate feedback from students about understanding of material presented. Asking students questions during the lecture period or asking students to summarize what they learned at the conclusion of the lecture period are examples of CAT. Course assessment may be achieved by requiring students to complete an evaluation form at the conclusion of the course. Students should be asked to evaluate the effectiveness of teaching methods, content organization, course materials and supplies, and practice exercises. Competency-based assessment tools should:

- Link educational objectives to performance
- Measure learner's performance against actual pharmacy technician performance standards
- Require learners to assess, analyze, and integrate material, then apply to practical situations

Competencies

On completion of the educational period, pharmacy technicians should be able to demonstrate competence in the following areas:

- Prescription receipt and screening for completeness and accuracy
- Medication preparation in sterile and nonsterile environments
- Medication and supply distribution
- Purchasing of pharmaceuticals, supplies, and devices
- Inventory control methods of medication, equipment, and devices
- Insurance billing and payment collection for medication and pharmacy services
- Pharmacy calculations necessary for prescription preparation, billing, and inventory control
- Federal and state regulations pertaining to receipt, sale, and dispensing of pharmaceuticals, as well as privacy regulations (Health Insurance Portability and Accountability Act of 1996 [HIPAA])
- Pharmacy equipment maintenance and use
- Pharmacy ethics
- Communicating effectively

Scope of Practice

According to the most recent Pharmacy Technician Certification Board Task Analysis (1998-1999), pharmacy technicians are performing tasks in three major categories: 64% report assisting the pharmacist in serving patients, 25% report that maintaining medication and inventory control systems is a core responsibility, and 11% are engaged in pharmacy practice management and administration. The majority of pharmacy technicians practice in community or hospital settings. The role of the pharmacy technician in managed care is expanding rapidly. Job descriptions for pharmacy technicians in community practice, hospital practice, and managed care are described in the next three sections.

Sample Pharmacy Technician Job Description—Community Pharmacy

General Definition

Under the direction of a pharmacist, the pharmacy technician performs pharmacy-related functions to facilitate the provision of optimal pharmaceutical care.

Responsibilities

- Help patients who are dropping off or picking up prescription orders
- Enter prescription orders into the computer
- Create a profile of the patient's health and insurance information in the computer or update the patient's profile
- Assist the pharmacist, under direct supervision, in the practice of pharmacy, in accordance with local, state, federal, and company regulations
- Communicate with insurance carriers to obtain payment for prescription claims
- At point of sale, verify that customer receives correct prescription(s)
- Order medications and supplies, place orders on shelves, and complete all associated paperwork
- Assist the pharmacist with filling and labeling prescriptions
- Prepare the pharmacy inventory
- Screen telephone calls for the pharmacist
- Communicate with prescribers and their agents to obtain refill authorization
- Compound oral solutions, ointments, and creams
- Prepackage bulk medications
- Assist in training new employees
- Assist other pharmacy technicians
- Assist pharmacist in scheduling and maintaining workflow

Sample Pharmacy Technician Job Description—Hospital Pharmacy

General Definition

Under the direction of a pharmacist, the pharmacy technician performs pharmacy-related functions, in compliance with sterile procedures and departmental policies, to provide optimal pharmaceutical care.

Responsibilities

- Rotate through all work areas of the pharmacy
- Transport medications, drug-delivery devices, and other pharmacy equipment from the pharmacy to nursing units and clinics

- Pick up copies of physician orders, automated medication administration records, and unused medications from the nursing units and return them to the pharmacy
- Fill patient medication cassettes
- Prepare medications and supplies for dispensing, including:
  - Prepacking bulk medications
  - Compounding ointments, creams, oral solutions, and other medicines
  - Preparing chemotherapeutic agents
  - Compounding total parenteral nutrition solutions
  - Compounding large-volume intravenous mixtures
  - Packaging and preparing drugs being used in clinical investigations
  - Preparing prescriptions for outpatients
  - Checking continuous unit dose medications
- Control and audit narcotics/stock substance
- Assist pharmacists in entering medication orders into the computer system
- Prepare inventories, order drugs and supplies from the storeroom, receive drugs and stock shelves in various pharmacy locations
- Screen telephone calls
- Perform monthly nursing unit inspections, maintain workload records, and collect quality-assurance data
- Assist in training new employees
- Assist other pharmacy technicians
- Coordinate insurance billing including third-party prescriptions
- Coordinate unit dose delivery
- Maintain and restock automated dispensing technology
- Triage telephone and window inquiries

Sample Pharmacy Technician Job Description—Managed Care

General Definition

Pharmacy technicians in managed care practice settings specialize in communicating with pharmacy benefit managers and resolving insurance billing issues. Skills required of managed care specialists may be used in all pharmacy practice settings.

Responsibilities

- Under the supervision of a pharmacist, daily handle on-going pharmacy benefit telephone calls from members, pharmacy providers, and physicians
- Troubleshoot third-party prescription claims questions with an understanding of on-line rejections and plan parameters
- Develop and maintain an electronic service log on all telephone calls with complete follow-up history
- Develop a trending report of the aforementioned service calls with an eye toward forecasting possible trends in pharmacy service
- Provide telephone and administrative support for the department as needed

Courses: Scope and Sequence

Certificate Program

Courses and Credit Hours for College-Based Pharmacy Technician Program (2 Semesters)

Essential Prerequisites

College English	3-5 credits
College Algebra or Business Math	3-5 credits
Keyboarding or Introduction to Computers	3-5 credits

Recommended Prerequisites

Chemistry	4-5 credits
Anatomy and Physiology	4-5 credits
Medical Terminology	3 credits

First Semester

Pharmacy Calculations	3 credits
Introduction to Pharmacy Practice	2 credits
Business and Professional Communication	3 credits
Pharmacology	3 credits
Pharmacy Record and Inventory Management	4 credits
Pharmacy Law and Ethics	2 credits
	17 credits

Second Semester

Pharmacology	3 credits
IV Admixture and Aseptic Technique	4 credits
Resumé Writing and Job Search	1 credit
Applied Pharmacy Technology	3 credits
AIDS Education and CPR	1 credit
Pharmacy Internship—Community Based*	3 credits
Pharmacy Internship—Institutional Based†	3 credits
	18 credits

Note: Correlation between contact hours and quarter/semester credits:
    One lecture hour = one credit (1:1)
    Two lab hours = one credit (2:1)
*Community internship: 200 hours
†Institutional internship: 200 hours

Courses and Credit Hours for College-Based Pharmacy Technician Program (3 Quarters)

First Quarter

Medical Vocabulary	3 credits
Orientation to Pharmacy Practice	2 credits
Pharmacy Calculations	3 credits
Communication Skills in Pharmacy	2 credits
Pharmacy Law	2 credits
Community Practice, Pharmacy Record and Inventory Management	4 credits
AIDS Education and CPR	1 credit
	17 credits

Second Quarter

Pharmacology I	3 credits
Over-the-Counter Drugs	2 credits
Applied Pharmacy Technology I	3 credits
IV Admixture and Aseptic Technique I	2 credits
Pharmacy Ethics	1 credit
Pharmacy Internship I*	4-6 credits
	15-17 credits

Third Quarter

Pharmacology II	3 credits
Applied Pharmacy Technology II	2 credits
IV Admixture and Aseptic Technique II	2 credits
Resumé Writing and Job-Finding Skills	1 credit
Insurance Billing	1 credit
Pharmacy Internship II†	7-9 credits
	16-18 credits

*On-the-job training in community and institutional care settings (hospital, home infusion, or long-term care)
†Total internship 13 credits (432 hours)

Courses for Modular Pharmacy Technician Program* (Clock Hours)

Core Learning Modules   (198 hr)

Module 1	Orientation to Pharmacy Practice	(22 hr)
Module 2	Pharmacy Calculations	(33 hr)
Module 3	Medical Terminology	(33 hr)
Module 8	Pharmacy Law	(33 hr)
Module 9	Pharmacology	(66 hr)
	(Treatment of Disorders of the Nervous System)	
	(Treatment of Disorders of the Skeletal-Muscular System)	
	(Treatment of Disorders of the Cardiovascular System)	
	(Treatment of Disorders of the Respiratory System)	
	(Treatment of Disorders of the Genitourinary System)	

*Adapted from *Model Curriculum for Pharmacy Technician Training,* ed 2, 2001 (view Model Curriculum for Pharmacy Technician Training at http://www.ashp.org/technician/model_curriculum/index.cfm?cfid=22856876&CFToken=60041269

	(Treatment of Disorders of the Gastrointestinal System)	
	(Treatment of Disorders of the Endocrine and Reproductive Systems)	
	(Treatment of Disorders of the Immune System)	
	(Treatment of Disorders of the Hematological System)	
	(Treatment of Disorders of the Skin and Eye, Ear, Nose, Throat)	
Module 10	Pharmacy Ethics	(11 hr)

Pharmacy Practice: Ambulatory Care Settings		**(296 hr)**
Module 4	Interpreting and Evaluating Prescriptions/Medication Orders	(22 hr)
Module 5	Prescription Preparation	(20 hr)
Module 6	Collecting and Recording Patient Data	(4 hr)
Module 7	Purchasing, Distribution and Inventory Control	(4 hr)
Module 12	Nonsterile Compounding	(16 hr)
Module 20	Pharmacy Internship, Community Practice	(230 hr)

Pharmacy Practice: Institutional Care Settings		**(296 hr)**
Module 11	Intravenous Admixture and Aseptic Technique	(66 hr)
Module 21	Pharmacy Internship, Institutional Practice	(230 hr)

Computer Use in Pharmacy Practice		**(55hr)**
Module 13	Computer Technology	(30 hr)
Module 14	Pharmacy Technician Role in Drug Utilization Review	(5 hr)
Module 15	Insurance Billing and Collection of Payment	(20 hr)

Other Essential Pharmacy Technician Courses		**(77 hr)**
Module 16	OTC Medications	(22 hr)
Module 17	Professional Organizations and Certification	(11 hr)
Module 18	Communication Skills in Pharmacy	(22 hr)
Module 19	Resumé Writing and Job-Finding Skills	(11 hr)
Module 22	AIDS Education and CPR	(11 hr)
		922 hr

Courses and Credit Hours for Associate of Applied Science Program (2 Years, 6 Quarters)

Essential Prerequisites

College Algebra or Business Math	3-5 credits
Keyboarding or Introduction to Computers	3-5 credits

First Year

First Quarter

College English	5 credits
Chemistry	3 credits
Anatomy and Physiology	3 credits
Medical Vocabulary	3 credits
Orientation to Pharmacy Practice	2 credits
	16 credits

Second Quarter

Pharmacy Calculations	3 credits
Community Practice, Pharmacy Record, and Inventory Mgmt	4 credits
Communication Skills in Pharmacy	3 credits
Pharmacology I	3 credits
Pharmacy Law	2 credits
	15 credits

Third Quarter

Pharmacy Ethics	1 credit
Pharmacology II	3 credits
Over-the-Counter Drugs	2 credits
Applied Pharmacy Technology I	3 credits
Pharmacy Internship I*	6 credits
	15 credits

Second Year

First Quarter

Microbiology	3 credits
IV Admixture and Aseptic Technique I	2 credits
AIDS Education	1 credit
Pharmacology II	3 credits
Applied Pharmacy Technology II	2 credits
Seminar: Advanced Insurance Billing	2 credits
	13 credits

Second Quarter

IV Admixture and Aseptic Technique II	2 credits
Seminar: Nonsterile Compounding	2 credits
Seminar: Pharmacy Technician Role in Drug Utilization Review	2 credits
Pharmacy Internship II†	7 credits
	13 credits

Third Quarter

Seminar: Supervisory and Management Skills for Pharmacy Technicians	2 credits
Seminar: Pharmacy Technician Role in Research and Data Collection	2 credits
Seminar: Nontraditional Practice Settings	2 credits
Resumé Writing and Job-Finding Skills	1 credit
Pharmacy Internship III‡	7 credits
	14 credits

---

*Pharmacy technician internship: community practice setting
†Pharmacy technician internship: institutional practice setting
‡Pharmacy technician internship: nontraditional practice setting

Degrees or Awards Conferred on Completion of Education Program

Pharmacy technician program graduates may be awarded a certificate of completion, diploma, or college degree (Associate of Applied Science degree) on successful completion of their education. College-based programs must satisfy State Board of Higher Education standards for granting certificates or Associates of Applied Science degrees. These usually require general education credits. These credits must often be obtained by taking specific general education courses such as psychology. It may be possible to substitute pharmacy technician program–required courses for the equivalent academic course. For example, Communication Skills in Pharmacy might satisfy the college human relations requirement and substitute for psychology. Alternatively, program directors should check to see if content "embedded" in pharmacy technician courses satisfy general education requirements.

Vocational and technical schools also have standards for granting certificates and diplomas. Program directors should consult state regulations, area employers, and their educational institution to determine which credential is mandatory or desirable in their area.

State and National Certification of Pharmacy Technicians

Some states require state or national certification of pharmacy technicians in addition to, or rather than, graduation from an accredited pharmacy technician program. Certification of competency for pharmacy technicians is currently awarded by either a State Board of Pharmacy or the Pharmacy Technician Certification Board (PTCB). PTCB is the only nationally recognized certification body. At present, more than 131,000 pharmacy technicians are PTCB certified. The current cost to sit for the PTCB certification exam is $120.00. Certification is valid for 2 years and requires 20 contact hours of pharmacy-related continuing education. The recertification cost for pharmacy technicians is $35.00.

Many State Boards of Pharmacy require registration, certification, or licensure of pharmacy technicians. Program directors should check their respective state board of pharmacy requirements and fees to appropriately advise pharmacy technician students. Websites for each State Board of Pharmacy is listed in the "State Boards of Pharmacy" section of this curriculum guide.

Course Descriptions/Sample Syllabi

Orientation to Pharmacy Practice

Course Description

This course reviews the contributions made by nations of the world to the practice of pharmacy, past and present. The course reviews the role of professional pharmacy organizations, past and present, in improving the practice of pharmacy and the role of the pharmacy personnel. Students also learn about new drug development, drug distribution, and the role of the pharmacy technician in drug procurement. Course material includes the types of sites that currently employ pharmacy technicians, including an analysis of the role of pharmacy technicians in various job settings. Current trends that may affect the future direction for pharmacy technicians, including national certification, are also discussed.

Course Outcomes/Learning Objectives

1. Describe the contributions made to the practice of pharmacy by nations of the world.
2. Identify selected pharmacy professional organizations and describe their functions.
3. Describe information resources available to pharmacy personnel and the role of the pharmacy technician in information collection.
4. Identify drug distribution centers and the role of the pharmacy technicians in drug procurement and distribution.
5. List health care providers who may prescribe and describe the limitations of their prescriptive authority.
6. List sites that employ pharmacy technicians and describe tasks of the pharmacy technician.
7. Describe current trends that may influence the practice of pharmacy and the future role of the pharmacy technician.
8. Describe the rationale for national certification of pharmacy technicians. Discuss the role of the Pharmacy Technician Certification Board and other organizations in this process.

Over-the-Counter Drugs

Course Description

This course reviews the use of nonprescription drugs for common disorders in which consumers seek advice for self-treatment. Students also learn questions to ask consumers that will help the pharmacist determine whether self-treatment is indicated or referral to medical care should be sought.

Course Outcomes/Learning Objectives

1. Define the term *non–legend drug*.
2. Compare and contrast the use and availability of non-legend drugs and legend drugs.
3. Describe common disorders in which consumers seek self-treatment.
   - Pain and inflammation
     a. Headache
     b. Osteoarthritis
     c. Menstrual cramps
     d. Canker sores
   - Fever
   - Motion sickness/nausea and vomiting
   - Insomnia
   - Allergic reactions
     a. Rashes/hives
     b. Eye allergies
     c. Hay fever
   - Cough and colds
     a. Congestion
     b. Rhinitis
     c. Cough
   - Fungal infections (topical)
     a. Jock itch
     b. Athlete's foot
     c. Vaginal infections
   - First aid
     a. Bites and stings
     b. Bacterial infection
     c. Burns
   - Acne
   - Lice and worms
   - Warts and calluses
   - Vitamins and herbals
4. Develop a list of questions that will help pharmacists determine the appropriateness of self-treatment.
5. For each classification of non–legend drugs covered, identify patient populations for whom usage is contraindicated or for whom cautious use is advised.
6. Learn common strengths, dosage forms, and directions for use of nonprescription medications used in the self-treatment of selected disorders.

Pharmacy Law

Course Description

This course is designed to introduce students to federal and state laws governing the practice of pharmacy. Special emphasis is given to areas of state laws regulating activities of pharmacy technicians.

Course Outcomes/Learning Objectives

1. Differentiate between responsibilities of pharmacy technician and pharmacist.
2. Differentiate between responsibilities of pharmacy technician and pharmacy assistant.

3. Identify penalties associated with failure to practice within scope.
4. Apply knowledge of state and federal law to dispense medication and maintain prescription records in compliance with state laws.
5. Demonstrate knowledge of product substitution laws in determination of product selection.
6. Apply knowledge of regulations pertaining to controlled substances to dispense medication and maintain prescription records in compliance with state laws.
7. Recognize errors of omission on hard copies.

Pharmacy Ethics

Course Description

This course explores commonly encountered ethical dilemmas from pharmacy practice. On completion of this course, students will have attained skills that will enable them to identify unethical behaviors, identify possible solutions, and analyze solutions for appropriateness using ethical decision-making models. Students learn evaluation skills that enable them to determine "the best possible solution" for a given ethical dilemma.

Course Outcomes/Learning Objectives

1. Describe models used in ethical decision making.
2. Use ethical decision-making models to identify ethical dilemmas in case presentations.
3. Analyze case presentations to determine possible solutions.
4. Prepare own case study using ethical decision-making models.
5. Evaluate potential effectiveness of solutions.
6. Learn to be receptive to arguments presented by classmates.
7. Provide feedback to classmates.
8. Assist in modification of plan for ethical resolutions.
9. Defend reasoning for plan of action.
10. Demonstrate consistent support for their positions.
11. Applications (case studies)
    - Cheating
    - Employee rights and obligations
    - Discrimination and stereotyping
    - Diversion
    - Ethical third-party billing
    - Accountability (taking responsibility for and reporting errors)
    - Valuing quality work
    - Codes of ethics

Pharmacology I

Course Description

This course reviews the principles of drug action including introduction to pharmacokinetics and pharmacodynamics. Students also study anatomy and physiology of the nervous system and discuss drugs used in the treatment of disorders of the nervous system.

Course Outcomes/Learning Objectives

1. Describe pharmacokinetic phases and give examples of factors influencing each phase.
2. Explain, using own words, drug receptor theory, and its relationship to dose response.
3. Describe anatomy and physiology of the nervous system.
4. Identify medications used in the treatment and disorders of the nervous system.

5. Demonstrate knowledge of warning label application for drugs used in treatment of disorders of the nervous system.
6. Identify important drug interactions that should be reported to pharmacist.
7. Learn common strengths, dosage forms, and directions for use of medications used in the treatment of disorders of the nervous system.

Topical Outline

I. Principles of Drug Action
II. Anatomy and Physiology of the Nervous System
III. Anatomy and Physiology of the Skeletal-Muscular System
IV. Treatment of Disorders of the Nervous System (classification of drugs, brand/generic names, therapeutic use, warning label usage, common strengths, and dosage forms)
   A. Anxiety
   B. Depression
   C. Psychosis
   D. Epilepsy
   E. Parkinson's disease
   F. Muscle spasm and other disorders
   G. Pain

Pharmacology II

Course Description

This course is a continuation of Pharmacology I. Students will briefly study the anatomy and physiology of the cardiovascular, gastrointestinal, endocrine, integumentary, respiratory, and reproductive systems. Students discuss treatment of bacterial and viral infections. Pharmacy technician role in the management of diabetes and hypertension is covered.

Course Outcomes/Learning Objectives

1. Describe anatomy and physiology of the cardiovascular, gastrointestinal, endocrine, reproductive, integumentary, and respiratory systems.
2. Identify medications used in the treatment of diseases of the cardiovascular, gastrointestinal, endocrine, integumentary, and respiratory systems.
3. Identify medications used in the treatment of selected bacterial and viral infections.
4. Demonstrate knowledge of warning label application for all drugs covered in Pharmacology II.
5. Identify important drug interactions that should be reported to the pharmacist.
6. Learn common strengths, dosage forms, and directions for use of all drugs covered in Pharmacology II.
7. Demonstrate knowledge and use of blood glucose and blood pressuring monitoring devices.

Topical Outline

I. Cardiovascular System
   A. Treatment of diseases of the cardiovascular system (classification of drugs, brand/generic names, therapeutic use, warning label usage, common strengths, and dosage forms)
      1. Angina
      2. Hypertension
      3. Myocardial infarction
      4. Arrhythmia
      5. Congestive heart failure
      6. Other

II. Gastrointestinal System
   A. Treatment of diseases of the gastrointestinal system (classification of drugs, brand/generic names, therapeutic use, warning label usage, common strengths, and dosage forms)
      1. Peptic ulcer disease
      2. Esophageal reflux
      3. Crohn's disease and ulcerative colitis
      4. Other
III. Endocrine and Reproductive System
   A. Treatment of diseases (classification of drugs, brand/generic names, therapeutic use, warning label usage, common strengths, and dosage forms)
      1. Hypothyroidism and hyperthyroidism
      2. Diabetes mellitus
      3. Paget's disease
      4. Hormone replacement therapy
      5. Contraception
      6. Addison's disease and Cushing's syndrome
      7. Other
IV. Respiratory System
   A. Treatment of diseases (classification of drugs, brand/generic names, therapeutic use, warning label usage, common strengths, and dosage forms)
      1. Asthma
      2. Chronic obstructive pulmonary disease
      3. Other
V. Treatment of Bacterial and Viral Infections
   A. Treatment of diseases (classification of antiinfectives and antivirals, brand/generic names, therapeutic use, warning label usage, common strengths, and dosage forms)
      1. HIV/AIDS
      2. Influenza
      3. Urinary tract infection
      4. Upper respiratory infection
      5. Other infections
VI. Integumentary System
   A. Acute & chronic skin disorders
   B. Use of corticosteroids & other agents to ameliorate skin disorders

Pharmacy Technology I

Course Description

This course reviews the history of computers in pharmacy, current practice applications, and future trends. Legal and ethical issues surrounding information collection and retrieval are also addressed. The laboratory component of this course is designed to provide students with skills and knowledge needed to process prescriptions using pharmacy software. Students will gain proficiency in the use of ambulatory care prescription processing software.

Course Outcomes/Learning Objectives

1. Describe application software and its usage in pharmacy settings.
2. Describe patient, political, and industry factors responsible for the expansion of the role of computers in the practice of pharmacy.
3. Describe use of computers in inventory control.
4. Describe use of computers in medication order entry.
5. Describe use of computers in quality assurance.
6. Compare uses of computers in ambulatory care and in-patient settings.

7. Demonstrate ability to use pharmacy software to process prescriptions.
8. Demonstrate ability to use pharmacy software for third-party claims adjudication.

Topical Outline

I. Computers in Pharmacy
   A. Ambulatory care
      1. Order entry
      2. Patient profiling
      3. Drug therapy monitoring
      4. Drug utilization review
      5. Inventory control
      6. Patient education
      7. Third-party claims adjudication
   B. In-patient (hospital, nursing home, home health care)
      1. Order entry
      2. Patient profiling
      3. Inventory control
      4. Drug distribution
      5. Medication administration records
      6. Quality assurance
      7. Bulk compounding
II. Prescription Processing
   A. Creating patient profiles
   B. Creating doctor files
   C. Creating drug files
   D. Creating caution messages
   E. Creating directions
   F. Creating prescription labels
   G. Insurance billing

Pharmacy Technology II

Course Description

This course reinforces what was learned in Pharmacy Technology I—specifically, prescription entry and billing to the third party. Students will gain a better understanding of insurance billing for prescriptions such as how to get correct information in order to avoid unnecessary problems. Additionally, students analyze rejected insurance claims to learn how to problem-solve billing issues and get the prescription "paid" by the insurance carrier. Students review patient profiling, prescription filling and refilling. Students will learn the use of dispense as written (DAW) codes, pneumonic direction (SIG) codes, prior authorization, denial overrides, and drug utilization review (DUR) codes. Additionally covered is merging and deleting files. Students in this course increase their knowledge of pharmaceuticals, learning approximately 100 additional drugs.

Course Outcomes/Learning Objectives

1. List brand names of drugs.
2. List generic names of drugs.
3. Select appropriate warning labels for drugs.
4. Classify drugs appropriately by therapeutic use.
5. Demonstrate ability to use pharmacy software to process prescriptions.
6. Demonstrate ability to accurately enter billing information into computer and generate billing reports.

Topical Outline

I. Drugs
   A. Uses
   B. Brand/generic names
   C. Warning labels
II. Computer Operations
   A. Ambulatory care
      1. Order entry
      2. Patient profiling
      3. Prescriber profiling
      4. Drug price updating
      5. Insurance billing and rebilling
      6. Handling insurance claims rejections
III. Prescription Processing
   A. Pouring and counting
   B. Prescription labeling
   C. Warning label usage

Pharmacy Calculations

Course Description

This course is a mathematics review with an introduction to calculations encountered in pharmacy practice.

Course Outcomes/Learning Objectives

1. Describe systems of weight, measure, and temperature used in pharmacy practice.
2. Accurately convert between apothecary, avoirdupois, metric, and household systems of measurement.
3. Identify common medication errors involving calculations.
4. Accurately compute
   - Percent concentrations
   - Drug dosages
   - Dilutions
   - Special care areas, for example, pediatric, intensive care
   - Formulas used to compound medicines
   - Volume or quantity to dispense
   - Number of days prescription will last (to determine eligibility for next refill)

Topical Outline

I. Basic Math Review
   A. Fractions: addition, subtraction, division, multiplication
   B. Decimals: addition, subtraction, division, multiplication
   C. Percents
   D. Ratios
   E. Converting values between each of the above four areas
   F. Roman numerals
II. Converting Between Measurement Systems
   A. Apothecary
   B. Metric
   C. Household

  III. Interpreting
     A. Prescriptions
     B. Physician orders
     C. Drug labels
  IV. Dosage Calculation Methods
     A. Ratio/proportion
     B. Formula method
     C. Alligation method
   V. Various Dosage Calculations
     A. Solids
     B. Liquids
     C. Powdered drugs
     D. Percent preparations
     E. Dilutions
     F. Compounding formulas
  VI. Calculations in Special Care Areas
     A. Pediatrics
     B. Intensive care

AIDS Education and CPR

Course Description

This course satisfies requirements for AIDS education for pharmacy technicians. Covered in the course is etiology of HIV/AIDS, universal precautions, and legal and ethical issues associated with HIV/AIDS. Students are exposed to psychosocial issues, and the global impact of the disease is presented. The role of the pharmacy technician, including Health Insurance Portability and Accountability Act of 1996 (HIPAA) regulations, is presented. American Heart Association guidelines for CPR are described, with opportunity for students to demonstrate an ability to perform according to standards.

Communication Skills for Pharmacy Practice

Course Description

This course is designed to assist students in developing the necessary communication skills to function competently as a contributing member in a pharmacy work setting. Students participate in team-building exercises and are introduced to effective communication tools. Furthermore, students learn skills to deal constructively with patients, information, ideas, and emotions associated with issues of diversity, culture, ethnicity, race, gender, religion, age, sexual orientation, and abilities.

Course Outcomes/Learning Objectives

1. Identify the developmental process of an effectively functioning staff.
2. Participate in team-building activities that strengthen staff cohesiveness.
3. Identify characteristics of cognitive, social, and moral development.
4. Develop effective and assertive staff communication skills.
5. Identify a variety of appropriate conflict management strategies.
6. Recognize the effects of change and stress on individuals.

Topical Outline

   I. Orientation and Group Processes
  II. Interpersonal Communication
 III. Perceptions and Communication
 IV. Social and Moral Development, Behaviorist Theory

V. Valuing Diversity
VI. Nonverbal Communication in Pharmacy
VII. Barriers to Communication
VIII. Listening and Empathetic Responding
IX. Assertiveness
X. Communicating Nondefensively
XI. Resolving Conflict
XII. Building Better Patient Understanding
XIII. Telephone Skills in Pharmacy
XIV. Special Situations

Community Practice, Pharmacy Records, and Inventory Management

Course Description

This course is designed to provide skills necessary to effectively practice in an ambulatory care setting. Students learn to interpret prescription contents, the top 100 drugs, inventory control procedures, tasks associated with procurement of pharmaceuticals, completing and filing records for third-party reimbursement, and requirements for completing and filing prescription records. Students are introduced to nonsterile compounding.

Course Outcomes/Learning Objectives

1. Able to accurately produce prescription labels at a rate consistent with industry standards.
2. Working knowledge of the forms commonly used in an ambulatory care practice setting; can select and accurately complete appropriate form for task.
3. Know brand and generic names of at least top 100 drugs.
4. Able to apply pharmacy calculations to accurately prepare and dispense pharmaceuticals.
5. Able to accurately select appropriate warning labels for top 100 drugs.
6. Able to recognize errors of omission on hardcopies.
7. Able to apply knowledge of pharmacy law to satisfy record keeping requirements and protect patient rights.
8. Demonstrate ability to compound selected prescriptions according to formula.

Topical Outline

I. Prescription Order Processing
  A. Patient data collection
    1. Patient profiling
    2. Confidentiality (HIPAA)
  B. Prescription content interpretation
    1. Interpretation of Latin abbreviations
    2. Prescription hard copy minimum requirements
  C. Application of pharmaceutical calculations
    1. Metric system
    2. Apothecary system
    3. Household equivalents
    4. Computation of quantity to dispense, days supply
  D. Introduction of dosage forms
    1. Methods of usage/application
  E. Application of prescription labeling requirements
    1. Label format
    2. Label data requirement

   II. Top 100 Drugs
      A. Generic to brand recognition
      B. Brand to generic recognition
      C. Therapeutic use
      D. Warning label usage
  III. Computer Skills
      A. Speed building
      B. Accuracy building
  IV. Third-Party Insurance Processing
      A. Form recognition
      B. General and specific plan billing limitations
      C. Common acronyms

IV Admixture and Aseptic Technique I

Course Description

This course is an introduction to aseptic techniques and sterile product preparation in institutional care settings. The devices and manipulation techniques necessary to maintain sterility and mechanics of a hospital pharmacy are discussed and practiced in laboratory exercises.

Course Outcomes/Learning Objectives

1. Introduce the student to sterile products and aseptic techniques.
2. Apply correct terminology and pharmacy calculations.
3. Learn IV systems, solutions and medications, including reconstitution of IV medications and expiration dates.
4. Know data entry, labeling, and profiling of pharmacy medications.
5. Demonstrate aseptic techniques and procedures in the laboratory setting.
6. Know theory and be able to demonstrate the use of laminar air flow (LAF) hood production of parenteral products.

Topical Outline and/or Major Divisions

    I. Proper Labeling
      A. Unit dose
      B. Expiration dates
   II. Intravenous Solutions
      A. LVP and minis
      B. Electrolytes
      C. Compatibilities
      D. Drugs
  III. Intravenous Devices
      A. Containers
      B. Tubing
      C. Needles
      D. Syringes
      E. Filters
      F. Pumps and regulators
      G. Ampoules and vials
      H. Heparin locks
      I. Central and peripheral catheters

IV. Aseptic Techniques
   A. Hand washing and touch contamination
   B. LAF hood technique and use
   C. Airborne contamination
   D. Transfer of solutions

IV Admixture and Aseptic Technique II

Course Description

A continuation of IV Admixture and Aseptic Technique I, IV Admixture and Aseptic Technique II focuses on the preparation of cardiac and other titerable drips, IV antibiotics, chemotherapy, large volume parenterals (LVP), and total parenteral nutrition (TPN). Students learn the basic indications and mechanism of actions of specific cardiac drugs, as well as calculations for selected drug concentrations. Proper technique for mixing and labeling thrombolytic, cardiac drips, and chemotherapeutic drugs is introduced. Laboratory sessions provide the opportunity for students to practice technique.

Course Outcomes/Learning Objectives

Introduce the rationale and development of TPN, chemotherapy, and intermittent infusion administration policies.
   1. Demonstrate proper technique for mixing and labeling thrombolytic drugs.
   2. Demonstrate proper technique for mixing and labeling cardiac drips.
   3. Understand the basic indications, mechanism of action, and specific drugs in the cardiac class.
   4. Calculate for specific drug concentrations, drip rates, and volume of cardiac medications needed for mixing.
   5. Demonstrate proper technique for mixing and labeling chemotherapy.
   6. Understand the basic indications, mechanism of action, and specific drugs in the chemotherapy class.
   7. Demonstrate proper technique for mixing and labeling TPNs.
   8. Understand the basic indications, mechanism of action, and specific drugs used for TPNs.
   9. Calculate for specific drug concentrations and fluid volumes of drugs needed to mix a TPN.
   10. Understand basic mixing and labeling requirements for compounded items.

Topical Outline

   I. TPN and Chemotherapy
      A. Types of TPN solutions
      B. Uses of TPN
      C. Types of additives
      D. Precautions in preparing chemotherapy
         1. Vertical flow hoods
         2. Disposal techniques
   II. Cardiac Drips
   III. Thrombolytics
   IV. Antibiotics
   V. Practical Considerations
      A. Labeling
      B. Drip rates
      C. Dosages calculations

Resumé Writing and Interview Techniques

Course Description

The goal of this course is to provide students with skills needed to seek and gain employment as a pharmacy technician. Students will learn how to write a cover letter and resumé. They will learn and practice interviewing techniques. Furthermore, students will learn strategies for job searching.

Course Outcomes/Learning Objectives

1. Prepare a resumé for employment.
2. Identify resources for locating job opportunities.
3. Describe interview strategies and practice interview techniques.

Advanced Insurance Billing

Course Description

This course covers third-party insurance plans and billing not previously covered in other courses. It includes plan limitations and strategies for solving billing issues. Students are provided a packet with pictures of various insurance cards and prescriptions so they can learn to recognize insurance carrier and practice entering insurance information, needed for claims adjudication, into patient profiles. Emphasis is on completing claims forms and problem-solving claims adjudication problems.

Course Outcomes/Learning Objectives

1. Obtain practical experience, knowledge, and skills to enable student to gain proficiency in claims adjudication.
2. Use problem-solving skills to develop solutions to billing problems.
3. Demonstrate ability to monitor and evaluate own performance (search for and correct mistakes).
4. Develop speed and accuracy and thus meet employer expectations of pharmacy technicians.

Pharmacy Technician Role in Drug Utilization Review

Course Description

This seminar course is designed to explore the role of the pharmacy technician in drug utilization review (DUR). The importance of patient profiles in the DUR process is explored, as is the role of the pharmacy technician in accurate and complete data collection and data entry into patient profiles. Also covered is the role of the pharmacy technician in assisting the pharmacist in screening for drug interactions, drug-disease state contraindications, drug allergies, and therapeutic duplication.

Course Outcomes/Learning Objectives

1. Describe pharmacy technician role in DUR.
2. Demonstrate ability to collect appropriate patient data and accurately create a patient profile.
3. Demonstrate ability to correctly identify drug interactions, therapeutic duplication, drug-allergy contraindications, and drug-disease state contraindications.
4. Demonstrate ability to appropriately respond to DUR computer-assisted screening messages and refer to appropriate level of authority.

Supervisory and Management Skills for Pharmacy Technicians

Course Description

Current and future practice requires pharmacy technicians to perform management or supervisory duties. This course is designed to prepare students to successfully assume managerial responsibilities.

Course Outcomes/Learning Objectives

1. Identify the developmental process of an effectively functioning staff.
2. Participate in team-building activities that strengthen staff cohesiveness.
3. Develop effective and assertive staff communication skills.
4. Identify a variety of appropriate conflict management strategies.

Pharmacy Technician Role in Research and Data Collection

Course Description

Pharmacy technicians may be required to engage in research activities in all practice settings. This course explores the role of pharmacy technicians in collecting and storing information associated with inventory procurement, clinical drug trials, drug information, poison prevention, and claims adjudication. This course introduces students to references for drug information found in most pharmacies and to pharmacy/medical databases. Resources for comparison and procurement of pharmaceuticals and supplies are also covered.

Course Outcomes/Learning Objectives

1. List sources for drug information.
2. List sources for pharmaceuticals and supply procurement.
3. Identify databases for drug information.
4. Describe the pharmacy technician role in research and data collection.

Nonsterile Compounding Seminar

Course Description

Compounding is becoming a niche market for many pharmacies. Pharmacy technicians in this course develop skills in compounding a variety of formulations. Students will learn to prepare product in a variety of dosage forms including ointments, creams, suppositories, and suspensions for oral and topical use. Students will be introduced to the resources provided by Professional Compounding Corporation of America (PCCA).

Course Outcomes/Learning Objectives

1. Accurately compute amount of drug needed to compound product.
2. Demonstrate proper use and care of compounding equipment.
3. Demonstrate proper weighing and measurement technique.
4. Demonstrate appropriate product formulation techniques.
5. Identify potential drug incompatibility problems.

Nontraditional Practice Settings

Course Description

Although the majority of pharmacy technicians are employed in ambulatory care and institutional practice settings, opportunities for employment in nontraditional practice settings are expanding. In this overview course, students are introduced to alternative pharmacy practice settings. Nontraditional pharmacy practice settings include mail order pharmacy, managed care, long-term care, home infusion, nuclear pharmacy, online pharmacy, and other practice settings.

Course Outcomes/Learning Objectives

1. Describe each nontraditional pharmacy practice setting.
2. Identify the role of the pharmacy technician in each nontraditional practice setting.

Pharmacy Internship I: Community Practice Settings

Course Description

The pharmacy technician internship is designed to enable students to obtain hands-on experience in a pharmacy setting. The primary objective of internship is to be sure the student gains practical experience, knowledge, skills, and insight into the various aspects of the pharmacy technician job. It is structured to be a learning experience, so the student and preceptor/teaching personnel should commit themselves to working toward that objective. This internship brings together all of the academic knowledge gained in the classroom with practical hands-on participation in various pharmacy settings. The clinical experience gained at these sites is invaluable in ensuring that the student becomes a competent pharmacy technician in all settings. Evaluation forms for both the student and preceptor must be completed separately.

Ambulatory care settings include chain pharmacy, independent pharmacy, and outpatient hospital/clinic pharmacy.

Course Outcomes/Learning Objectives

1. Obtain practical experience, knowledge, and skills to enable student to gain proficiency in a structured learning environment.
2. Learn employer expectations of pharmacy technician.
3. Develop work ethic skills.
4. Perform duties of a pharmacy technician in an ambulatory care pharmacy setting.

Pharmacy Internship II: Institutional Care Settings

Course Description

Pharmacy Technician Internship II is similar to the Community Practice externship except that students are exposed to pharmacy practice in an institutional care setting. The primary objective of internship is to be sure the student gains practical experience, knowledge, skills, and insight into the various aspects of the pharmacy technician job in a structured learning environment. This internship brings together all of the academic knowledge gained in the classroom, with an emphasis on aseptic technique and sterile product preparation. Evaluation forms for both the student and preceptor must be completed separately.

Inpatient settings include nursing home, inpatient hospital, and home infusion.

Course Outcomes/Learning Objectives

1. Obtain practical experience, knowledge, and skills to enable student to gain proficiency in a structured learning environment.
2. Learn employer expectations of pharmacy technician.
3. Develop work ethic skills.
4. Perform duties of a pharmacy technician in an institutional care pharmacy setting.

Pharmacy Internship III: Nontraditional Pharmacy Practice

Course Description

Pharmacy Technician Internship III is similar to the Community and Institutional Practice Externship except that students are exposed to nontraditional pharmacy practice settings. Nontraditional pharmacy practice settings include mail order pharmacy, managed care insurance claims specialist, long-term care, home health, nuclear pharmacy, on-line pharmacy, pharmacy software customer care specialist, and other pharmacy practices.

The primary objective of internship is to be sure the student gains practical experience, knowledge, skills, and insight into the various aspects of the pharmacy technician job in a structured learning environment. This internship brings together all of the academic knowledge gained in the classroom, with an emphasis on aseptic technique and sterile product preparation. Evaluation forms for both the student and preceptor must be completed separately.

Instructional Methods

A wide variety of instructional methods may be used to facilitate student learning. The modality that the instructor selects should engage students, enhance understanding of concepts, and enable students to practice skills. A combination of lecture and laboratory is critical to a successful vocational education program. Labs are designed to enable students to practice skills under the guidance of a skilled practitioner before using these skills in a real practice setting. It is appropriate to use a variety of teaching modalities throughout the educational training period. All of the following methods have been used in pharmacy technician programs.

- On-campus lecture
- On-campus lab
- E-mail
- Asynchronous web conference
- Broadcast telecourse
- On-line course
- Computer
- Two-way interactive classroom
- Videocassette
- Other (please specify):

Program designers should determine the number of contact hours to be assigned to each instructional method.

Classroom Learning Strategies

Lecture

Lecture is the most commonly used instructional method; however, it has many limitations. It is the most passive method of learning and offers limited opportunity to assess student attainment of knowledge. Classroom assessment techniques such as frequent questioning of students can assist the instructor in determining student understanding of key concepts.

Lecture is most effective when the instructor cites examples from actual practice to demonstrate applicability of material. Although many students prefer lecture to mirror textbook readings, more is gained by presentation of material not found in the required text but based on text readings. Pharmacy technicians and pharmacists currently employed in pharmacy practice settings can contribute valuable "real life" experience and enhance the effectiveness of this teaching method.

When using lecture as an instructional method, consider ways in which students learn. Students may be auditory, visual, or kinesthetic learners. Students learn only 70% of the content by any single instructional method. Multiple instructional methods must be used to enable students to learn 100% of the content. Lectures accommodate the auditory learner at the expense of visual and kinesthetic learners. The use of visual aids, writing information on white or blackboards, and/or use of overhead projectors can significantly enhance the lecture-learning experience.

Lecture is an appropriate instructional method for some, but not all, pharmacy technician courses. Courses where this method has been used satisfactorily are pharmacy law, orientation to pharmacy practice, medical vocabulary, pharmacology, and nonprescription medicines.

Video

Videos may be used successfully to enhance the educational experience. They bring the expertise of other professionals into the classroom. Videos may be used along with lecture and demonstration to show graphically how to perform a specific task or procedure.

It is helpful to develop a list of learning objectives for each video. These objectives are presented before showing the video so that learners can focus on key video points. Immediately after the video, learners should be questioned to ascertain whether key concepts were grasped. It may also be useful to start and stop videos at appropriate times and engage students in discussion of key concepts.

Videos are an important component of the multimedia learning environment. Although they are essentially like a lecture, the visuals and entertainment value enhance the learning experience.

Pharmacy technician courses enhanced by the use of video instruction include Orientation to Pharmacy Practice, Pharmacology, Pharmacy Ethics, Pharmacy Technology, Sterile Products and Aseptic Technique, and Communication Skills in Pharmacy Practice.

Computer

Computer-aided instruction is becoming increasingly popular. Currently available software enables instructors to create lectures and demonstrations that are visually stimulating to today's student. The creative lecturer can use PowerPoint and other software to create lecture material. Video clips can be embedded in a slide show to create a true multimedia presentation. Slides can be printed and given to students for study notes.

Because pharmacy technicians perform increasingly more tasks with the assistance of computers, it is important for them to be literate and familiar with the use of area pharmacy-based software. Pharmacy-based software enables students to process and label prescriptions. If the pharmacy technician program has a designated computer lab, open labs can be scheduled that permit students to gain extra prescription processing practice. Most prescription processing software is proprietary and requires large memory reserves; thus it cannot be downloaded onto students' personal computers. Software is available for prescription processing and creating labels in institutional and ambulatory care settings. Examples of software are listed in the chapter titled Resources and Supplies.

Interactive software designed for students to learn and study core concepts is also available. Many pharmacology, pharmacy calculations, and medical vocabulary texts come with a CD ROM disk. This software facilitates self-paced instruction. Students can review material or practice skills at their own pace.

The Internet is an important tool and is used to facilitate student self-discovery. Chapter 6 of *Mosby's Pharmacy Technician Principles and Practice*, Referencing, is devoted to the importance of research skills for pharmacy technicians. To develop these skills, pharmacy technician instructors can design Internet research assignments. The Internet is saturated with information, not all of which is scientifically valid. It is important to teach students how to evaluate Internet content, as well as where to locate desired information. It is equally important to discuss plagiarism and intellectual property rights with students so that they will understand the ethical and legal implications of "cutting and pasting" information found on the Internet into their assignments.

Demonstration

Demonstration is an effective teaching method, especially when followed immediately by opportunity for student practice. A variety of methods may be used to demonstrate skill and core concepts or model behaviors. Instructors may gather small groups of students and perform the skill, show a video, or use a data projector to demonstrate to a large group.

Demonstrations always precede student labs to show learners how to perform tasks correctly. It is important to demonstrate prescription processing, insurance billing, prescription preparation and filling, aseptic technique, and pharmacy calculations. It is also important to model appropriate and ethical interaction between pharmacy technician, patient care providers, and patients.

Instructors using this valuable instructional method must remember to dissect complex processes into small parts and then demonstrate each part in the order in which it will be performed. Adequate time to practice each step must be permitted if learners are to become proficient in performing the skill.

Lab Assignments

Labs provide learners the opportunity to practice the skills they have been taught in a supportive and controlled learning environment under the guidance of experienced professionals and instructors. Hands-on practice is the instructional method most conducive to competency-based education. In the classroom the pharmacy technician learner is shown how to process prescriptions using pharmacy-based software. The same student is provided a list of important patient data to collect in order to properly process a prescription. In lab, the student is presented a prescription and must demonstrate she/he is able to gather the necessary information from the patient, then using the pharmacy software accurately process the prescription.

Labs should be designed using the competency-based curriculum model. Lab exercises should be built on actual pharmacy technician performance expectations and simulate actual work-related situations. Repetition is key to attainment of learning objectives. By having students partner with each other to check each other's lab assignments, opportunities are created for learners to work with and learn from each other, as well as learn to evaluate their performance and the work of others. Integrate pharmacy students into pharmacy technician labs, if possible, to further simulate a real-world experience. This benefits both the pharmacist in-training and the pharmacy technician in-training. As learning progresses, lab exercises should become increasingly more complex and challenging, thus enabling learners think critically, problem-solve, and develop solutions. A lab manual, with all learning exercises, should be created. The lab manual should identify skills students are expected to attain by the conclusion of the experiential training period.

Lab assessment tools should be designed to:

1. Measure learner's performance against actual pharmacy technician performance standards
2. Require learners to assess, analyze, and integrate material then apply to practical situations

Independent Study

Independent study projects help students gain information not presented in the classroom. Another goal is to encourage student development into lifelong learners. Pharmacy technician is a profession that requires continued education beyond the initial training period. New medications, third-party insurance, prescription processing software, and technology are continually being introduced. Current educational models place the instructor in the role of facilitator of student self-learning, rather than the person that "pours knowledge into the student," thus the change from teacher/student to facilitator/learner.

Independent study can be designed as an individual or group learning experience. Group study encourages students to learn from each other and encourages team building. In pharmacy practice the pharmacy technicians and pharmacist must work as a team to provide the best pharmaceutical care to patients.

Small Group Discussions

Small group discussion can be used in conjunction with independent study, lecture, or labs. Small groups of four to eight learners are most effective. As with group independent study, small group instruction requires student collaboration. Collaboration on case studies, problem-solving activities, and text or instructor-designed exercises gets students sharing ideas and evaluating information, thereby creating a dynamic learning environment.

Immediately after presentation of information by the lecturer, students might be instructed to break into small groups to discuss a related case. By listening to group discussions, the lecturer can assess the student's ability to analyze and synthesize information presented. Furthermore, the pharmacy technician lecturer should monitor discussions and presentations for accuracy and contribute additional information as needed. Students that are able to teach others and/or discuss concepts in small groups often demonstrate a greater depth of understanding. In fact, this method of assessing student's abilities may be superior to examination.

It is recommended that the pharmacy technician instructor create student groups rather than let students form their own groups. This enables the instructor to create groups that pair vocal with quiet students and strong students with those that need additional help, and to discourage cliques in favor of interacting with the diverse student body. Additional guidelines for group work are:

- All learners must participate in discussions.
- All learners must contribute to material presented (when an oral presentation is required).

The amount of time devoted to group collaboration varies; however, 30 to 45 minutes is adequate for most small group discussions. Less time limits the discussion, but if too much time is allotted, students may begin to discuss topics unrelated to the learning material. Peer evaluation of group projects, if used properly, can be a valuable learning tool.

Pharmacy technician courses that are enhanced by this instructional method include Pharmacy Ethics, Communication Skills in Pharmacy Practice, Pharmacology, Pharmacy Calculations, Pharmacy Law, and Orientation to Pharmacy Practice.

Distance Learning

Educational institutions are increasingly exploring distance learning as a method for pharmacy technician education. Distance learning instructional methods include online classrooms, synchronous or asynchronous web conferencing, two-way (or more) interactive classrooms, broadcast telecourses, video, and e-mail. These educational modalities provide a means to get formal education through an accredited institution to students who do not live within commutable distance to the academic institution.

Course content traditionally imparted via a traditional lecture format is easily tailored to a distance-learning format, and if labs are supervised by an assistant on site, synchronous web conferencing may be appropriate for laboratory courses. Regardless of the primary method of instruction, pharmacy technician programs must provide students the opportunity for on-the-job experiences.

Midlands Technical College in Columbia, South Carolina, embarked on a project to provide pharmacy technician training to underserved areas in rural South Carolina, which would include an organized laboratory experience with hands-on activities.* South Carolina Educational Television Network was selected by Midlands Technical College to deliver live satellite broadcasts of lectures. Two sites geographically accessible to students were established for hands-on laboratory experiences. Both lectures and laboratory sessions were designed by using real-time technology so that students could ask questions and their performance could be observed. On-the-job experiences were obtained at pharmacy sites within a reasonable commutable distance for students. Results of this method of educating pharmacy technicians showed little difference in grade point averages of students trained on campus at Midlands Technical College and distance-learning students.†

Pharmacy technician education via distance learning can be found in institutions from North Dakota (North Dakota State College of Science) to Texas. All of these programs build in on-the-job training.

Distance learning poses some challenges. Course offered via videocassette lack spontaneous interaction between learner and instructor. Student-lecturer and student-student interaction is limited, even when synchronous web conferencing or interactive classrooms are used. If technology used to link classrooms together is voice activated, cameras will be directed to the classroom where the first voices are heard. Verbal exchange by students speaking at other sites will not be heard. To avoid background noise, table microphones typically are turned off until a question is asked, which also may limit spontaneity. Courses taught online are best when a real-time "chat room" is established to facilitate communication among students. Care must be taken to ensure that the student completing coursework and exams is the student registered for the course.

Pharmacy technician courses that are amenable to this instructional method include Pharmacology, Pharmacy Calculations, Pharmacy Law, Over-the-Counter Drugs, and Orientation to Pharmacy Practice.

Homework

Homework, when assigned before class discussion, prepares students to actively participate in class activities. A well-prepared student is more apt to engage in class discussion, comes to class with questions about text readings, and is able to concentrate on what is being presented rather than furiously writing notes.

---

*Ballington D. Hammett S: Training pharmacy technicians in support of rural health initiatives: a South Carolina experience, *J Pharm Technol* 15:177, 1999.
†Ibid., p. 180.

Student Clinics

Tutorial sessions run by instructor or student are a useful method to reinforce or clarify information provided. Clinics should be scheduled on a regular basis. Student-run clinics can help develop leadership skills and help to develop critical thinking skills.

Field Trips

Visits to practice settings, drug distribution centers, and board of pharmacy open meetings are useful methods to demonstrate application of skills or concepts discussed in the classroom. Field trips are also a great way to promote your pharmacy technician program and establish working relationships with area employers and state boards of pharmacy.

Experiential Learning Strategies

Experiential learning can be obtained in classroom laboratories, as well as in actual pharmacy practice settings. Both are critical to the education of pharmacy technicians. Classroom lab instruction was discussed previously (see Lab Assignments, pp 28-29); here we discuss the need for experiential learning in a pharmacy practice setting.

Ideally, students should be exposed to as many practice settings as possible. At minimum students should gain extensive experience in a community practice setting and an institutional practice setting.

It is essential to develop an experiential training manual for pharmacy technician experiential learning. A training manual is useful to preceptors as it identifies skills students should learn/practice during the training period. Students should also be evaluated on attainment of personal attributes essential to effective and efficient performance as a pharmacy technician. A good experiential training manual also includes information that will help the pharmacist or technician trainer become a more effective educator. An experiential training manual assists students by identifying skills they are expected to attain by the conclusion of the experiential training period.

The experiential training manual should include a summary of what is to be gained from experiential learning, as well as all performance evaluation tools and a record of hours spent in training. In addition to evaluation forms completed by the student's preceptor, instructors can evaluate student progress and appropriateness of learning activities through student journaling. Furthermore, the experiential training manual should include form(s) for students to evaluate the training site. Just as students benefit from constructive feedback, trainers benefit from students' evaluation of their training.

Experiential learning evaluations should:

1. Include direct observation
2. Assess skills attainment using a proficiency rating scale
3. Assess learner attitude and responsibility for work performed
4. Peer and self-assessment

Sample competency rating scale I

1. Demonstrates outstanding potential
2. Exceeds minimum potential
3. Meets minimum potential
4. Fails to meet minimum potential

Sample competency rating scale II

1. Skilled, can work independently
2. Moderately skilled, needs limited supervision
3. Limited skills, requires instruction and close supervision
4. No experience in this area

Experiential training sites should be selected according to training experience offered and commitment by the pharmacist and pharmacy technicians to train student learners. It is highly recommended that the pharmacy technician program discuss training expectations with the pharmacy internship site and the student. An affiliation agreement between training site and pharmacy technician program is frequently required. Affiliation agreements should include a list of program expectations of the training site and a list of site expectations of the program. These agreements typically cover topics such as:

1. Minimum educational requirements before beginning internship (e.g., HIPAA training, aseptic technique)
2. Standards for educational achievement before students are permitted to begin internship
3. Requirements for supervision of students at training site
4. Joint responsibility for evaluation of students
5. Liability coverage

Affiliation agreements are legally binding. Thus they must be reviewed by Human Resources, the pharmacy, and the pharmacy technician program counsel.

Community Service Learning

Service learning can provide a valuable learning experience for the pharmacy technician student, as well as benefit the community. It also provides great exposure for the pharmacy technician program. Opportunities for service learning could include giving poison prevention workshops to preschoolers and their care providers or demonstrating the proper use of blood glucose and blood pressure monitors at senior centers. The only limit to this community service learning may be state restrictions on scope of practice for pharmacy technicians. Campus Compact is a national coalition of colleges and universities committed to infusion of civic purposes in education. Its website (http://www.compact.org/) provides instructions on where to get grants to design curriculum that incorporates community service. Students may obtain "Learn-and-Serve" fellowships, too.

Program Assessment

Assessment is an ongoing process aimed at understanding and improving student learning. It involves making our expectations explicit and public; setting appropriate criteria and high standards for learning quality; systematically gathering, analyzing, and interpreting evidence to determine how well performance matches those expectations and standards; and using the resulting information to document, explain, and improve performance. When it is embedded effectively within larger institutional systems, assessment can help us focus our collective attention, examine our assumptions, and create a shared academic culture dedicated to ensuring and improving the quality of higher education.*

Program review benefits students, pharmacy technician programs, and institutions. When review results in a program that closely correlates with institutions' curricula, academically supports incoming student needs, leads to effective use of fiscal and human resources, students benefit. Ongoing program evaluation improves teaching and learning. Institutions benefit because outcome measures provide strategies for institutional problem solving and improvement.

The following are program-assessment questions:

1. Do program goals correspond to those of the institutional shared vision statement?
2. Are resources adequate to meet program needs?
3. Is the program meeting the needs of the community?
4. Are students achieving desired outcomes?
5. How will/do the method(s) of instruction affect specific course requirements such as labs, peer-to-peer interaction, or group discussion?
6. Does the program promote student success through instruction, programs, and services that are convenient, accessible, innovative, student-centered, and supported by effective use of technology?
7. Does the program foster a supportive community environment that promotes diversity and encourages each individual's best work and learning?
8. Are pharmacy employers, pharmacists, and pharmacy technicians involved in program assessment and determination of current employee needs? (Technical Advisory Committee [TAC], former grads, potential employers, pharmacy technicians, pharmacists, organized labor)
9. Does the program involve pharmacists, employers, and pharmacy technicians in determining future trends for pharmacy technicians?

*Angelo, Thomas, Reassessing (and Defining) Assessment, AAHE Bulletin 48(3): Nov. 1995.

Defining Program Success

Success of pharmacy technician programs is assessed by a variety of measures. These may include, but are not limited to, the following:

1. Student enrollment
2. Program completion rate (successful completion of all coursework and graduation)
3. Active waiting list for program
4. Number of graduates employed within 3 months after graduation
5. Requests by employers to become a placement site for student training
6. Demand for graduates—measured by employers who ask college to announce/post job openings to current and graduated students
7. Demonstration of attainment of skills through satisfactory completion of lab assignments
8. Satisfactory evaluations by externship supervisors

When evaluating program success, consider internal and external factors that influence the pharmacy technician program. Program enrollment is influenced by the reputation and quality of the pharmacy technician program, program cost, and availability of classes (internal factors). It is also influenced by the number of competing pharmacy technician programs, on-the-job training opportunities, job-market trends, and economic outlook (external factors).

Factors Influencing Student Outcomes

A variety of factors may influence student outcomes. The pharmacy technician program must recognize factors that interfere with student persistence and provide advice and support to students. These factors include:

- Course requirements
- Childcare needs, availability, and accessibility
- Outside employment
- On-the-job training programs
- Family support or lack of support
- Institutional support
- Inflexible course scheduling

Accrediting Standards for Pharmacy Technician Programs

Pharmacy technician programs are currently accredited by the American Society of Health Systems Pharmacists (ASHP), Accrediting Bureau of Health Education Schools (ABHES), Accrediting Council for Independent Colleges and Schools (ACICS), and individual state boards of pharmacy. In 2002, approximately 247 schools and training institutions offered pharmacy technician training. Credentials awarded included associate degree, certificate, and diploma. Additionally, ASHP accredits programs as do state boards of pharmacy. Accredited programs may be found in schools/institutions or be on-the-job training. Certification and board of pharmacy approval of pharmacy technician programs ensure that all graduates have a minimum level of competence. Certification demonstrates that those minimum competencies have been achieved. Program directors should consult state regulations, area employers, and their educational institution to determine which accreditation is mandatory or desirable in their area.

American Society of Health System Pharmacists

ASHP is one of the first organizations to establish standards for pharmacy technician training programs. Although only one state requires ASHP accreditation for pharmacy technician training programs, many programs nationwide have obtained ASHP accreditation. Currently ASHP standards require a minimum of 600 hours of contact time over a minimum period of 15 weeks. ASHP is currently the only accrediting body that has set a national training standard. Fees associated with ASHP accreditation are listed in the table on the next page. Additional information can be found at the ASHP website http://www.ashp.org/technician.

The annual accreditation fee combines both the annual fee and the site survey fee and spreads assessment in equal increments over the entire accreditation cycle.

Pharmacy Technician Training Programs

Program site(s)	Annual assessment 2003 (6-year cycle)	Annual assessment 2004 (6-year cycle)
1	$1,505	$1,600
2	$2,045	$2,150
3	$2,340	$2,475
4	$2,635	$2,775
5 or more	$2,935	$3,100

2003 initial application fee is $315 per technician program
2004 initial application fee is $325 per technician program
Note: The annual assessment fee and application fee are subject to change yearly.

Accrediting Bureau of Health Education Schools

The ABHES is listed as a nationally recognized accrediting agency by the U.S. Department of Education. ABHES accredits postsecondary institutions specializing in allied health education and specialized programs for medical assistants in the private sector and medical laboratory technicians in the public and private sectors. A complete list of fees can be found at the ABHES website http://www.abhes.org.

2003-2004 ABHES User Fees

User Fees (All Applications for Accreditation). *(Institutional, MA program, MLT program, Institutional, Non-main Campus, & Additional Classroom Location)*

Initial Applicant (first location)	$2,000
(each non-main campus)	$1,000
(includes change in status from programmatic to institutional)	
New Additional Classroom Location	$500
New Non-Main Campus Business Plan, Application, and Self-Evaluation	$2,000
New Program (first location)	$750
(each additional location)	$250
New Associate Degree program (first location)	$900

Accrediting Council for Independent Colleges and Schools

ACICS, a nonprofit education corporation, is recognized by the U.S. Secretary of Education as an independent and autonomous national accrediting body that accredits institutions of higher education offering programs of study through the master's degree level, including pharmacy technician programs. A complete listing of fees can be found on the ACICS website http://www.acics.org.

Application and other fees	Fee
Initial Grant (per main and branch)	$2,500
New Grant (Reevaluation, per main and branch)	$2,000*
Branch-to-Freestanding	$1,500*
Application to Initiate a Branch Campus	$2,500
Program Application (first location)	$1,000
Program Application (same program at other locations)	$500
Distance Education Application (first location)	$250
Distance Education Application (same program at other locations)	$175
Application to Initiate a Learning Site	$1,000
Fee for Late Submission	$500[†]
Special Visit Fee	$3,000

*Plus a $500 surcharge for each learning site and $250 for each specialized program.

[†] Late Fees will be charged for the late submission of an Annual Institutional Report, Annual Financial Report, self-study, payments, and other Council-directed submissions having a specific due date.

State Training Requirements

According to the American Council on Pharmaceutical Education (ACPE), 51% of states specify training requirements in their regulations. Thirty-nine percent (39%) require board review of the training and only one currently requires American Society of Health Systems Pharmacists (ASHP) accreditation of the training program.

As minimum requirements for pharmacy technician education and training vary, those wishing to establish pharmacy technician programs should contact the board of pharmacy in their state. Washington State Board of Pharmacy education and training requirements are shown here as an example of state regulations.

WAC 246-901-030 Technician Education and Training

(1) Pharmacy technicians must obtain education or training from one of the following:
    (a) Formal academic program for pharmacy technician training approved by the board.
    (b) On-the-job training program approved by the board.
(2) The minimum educational prerequisite for entering a training program shall be high school graduation or G.E.D.
(3) In order to receive certification as a pharmacy technician, the technician must send the board the following:
    (a) A state application indicating completion of board approved training program;
    (b) Proof of successful completion of a certification examination approved by the board.
(4) An out-of-state pharmacy technician applicant must meet the same requirements as a pharmacy technician trained in this state. The board must approve training programs approved in other states.
(5) Applicants whose academic training has been obtained in foreign countries shall meet certification requirements as listed below:
    (a) Foreign pharmacy school graduates. Board approval of program completed for the degree.
    (b) Foreign medical school graduates. Board approval of program completed for the degree.
    (c) All foreign graduates for whom English is not the primary language shall provide proof of receiving a score of at least 173 on the Test of English as a Foreign Language (TOEFL) and a score of 50 on the Test of Spoken English (TSE) prior to certification.
    (d) Foreign trained applicants must earn 520 hours of supervised experience in an approved pharmacy technician training program.
(6) Prior to performing specialized functions, pharmacy technicians shall complete specialized training and meet proficiency criteria set forth by the board.
    (a) Unit-dose medication checking. The training proficiency criteria requires demonstration of 99% accuracy in medication checking.
    (b) Intravenous admixture preparation. The training proficiency criteria requires demonstration of 100% accuracy in intravenous admixture preparation of a representative sample of preparations provided by the facility using aseptic technique.

[Statutory Authority: RCW 18.64.005, chapter 18.64A RCW. 00-15-081, § 246-901-030, filed 7/19/00, effective 8/19/00. Statutory Authority: RCW 18.64.050. 94-08-097, § 246-901-030, filed 4/6/94, effective 5/7/94. Statutory Authority: RCW 18.64.005 and chapter 18.64A RCW. 91-18-057 (Order 191B), recodified as § 246-901-030, filed 8/30/91, effective 9/30/91; Order 141, § 360-52-020, filed 12/9/77.]

WAC 246-901-035 Pharmacy Technician Specialized Functions

A pharmacy technician who meets established criteria for employment, experience, training and demonstrated proficiency may perform specialized functions. The criteria shall be specified in the utilization plan of the pharmacy for pharmacy technicians performing specialized functions required in WAC 246-901-100 (2)(b). Records of pharmacy technician training and of demonstration of proficiency shall be retrievable within 72 hours on request to the board. Specialized functions include the following:

(1) Unit-dose medication checking. Following verification of the drug order by a licensed pharmacist, a pharmacy technician may check unit-dose medication cassettes filled by another pharmacy technician or pharmacy intern in pharmacies serving facilities licensed under chapter 70.41, 71.12, 71A.20 or 74.42 RCW. No more than a forty-eight hour supply of drugs may be included in the patient medication cassettes and a licensed health professional must check the drug before administering it to the patient.

(2) Registration of pharmacy assistants. Any person desiring registration as a pharmacy assistant shall apply to the board for registration on forms to be supplied by the board. The fee for registration will be included in the fee for authorization to utilize the services of pharmacy ancillary personnel.

WAC 246-901-060 Technician Certification

To become certified as a pharmacy technician, an individual must:

(1) Complete an approved pharmacy technician program;

(2) Apply to the board for certification. The application must include a notarized statement of program verification signed by the program director.

It is the responsibility of the pharmacy technician to maintain a current mailing address with the board as required by chapter 246-12 WAC. Pharmacy technicians shall notify the board of any change of mailing address within 30 days of the change.

Websites for each state board of pharmacy are listed on pp. 42 and 43.

Resources for Accreditation Standards for Pharmacy Technician Programs and Credentialing of Pharmacy Technicians

Organization	Phone Number	Website
American Council on Pharmaceutical Education	(312) 664-3575 FAX: (312) 664-7008	http://www.acpe-accredit.org
Council on Credentialing in Pharmacy		http://www.pharmacycredentialing.org
Pharmacy Technician Educators Council	Telephone: (562) 860-1927 Ext 417	http://www.rxptec.org
National Association of Boards of Pharmacy	(847) 698-6227	http://www.nabp.net
American Society of Health Systems Pharmacists	(301) 657-3000	http://www.ashp.org
Pharmacy Technician Certification Board	(202) 429-7576 FAX: (202) 429-7596	http://www.ptcb.org
American Pharmaceutical Association	(202) 628-4410	http://www.aphanet.org
National Institute of Standards in Pharmacist Credentialing	(703) 299-8790 FAX: (703) 683-3619 E-mail: questions@nispcnet.org	http://www.nispcnet.org
National Association of Chain Drug Stores	(703) 549-3001	http://www.nacds.org

Continued

Organization	Phone Number	Website
American Association of Pharmacy Technicians	Bobbie Craddock (210) 297-7764 president@pharmacytechnician.com	http://www.pharmacytechnician.com
Accrediting Council for Independent Colleges and Schools	750 First Street, NE Suite 980 Washington, DC 20002-4241 TEL: (202) 336-6780 FAX: (202) 842-2593 E-mail:info@acics.org	http://www.acics.org/
Accrediting Bureau for Health Education Schools	ABHES 7777 Leesburg Pike, Suite 314 N. Falls Church, VA 22043 (703) 917-9503 FAX: (703) 917-4109 E-mail: info@abhes.org	http://www.abhes.org/
National Health Career Association	NHA-National Headquarters 134 Evergreen Place, 9th Floor East Orange, NJ 07018 Phone: (973) 678-9100 (800) 499-9092 FAX: (973) 678-7305	http://www.nhanow.com

State Boards of Pharmacy

Alabama State Board of Pharmacy
http://www.albop.com

Alaska Board of Pharmacy
http://www.dced.state.ak.us/occ//ppha.htm

Arizona State Board of Pharmacy
http://www.pharmacy.state.az.us

Arkansas State Board of Pharmacy
http://www.state.ar.us/asbp

California State Board of Pharmacy
http://www.pharmacy.ca.gov

Colorado State Board of Pharmacy
http://www.dora.state.co.us/pharmacy

Connecticut Commission of Pharmacy
http://www.ctdrugcontrol.com/rxcommision.htm

Delaware State Board of Pharmacy
http://professionallicensing.state.de.us/boards/pharmacy/index.shtml

District of Columbia Board of Pharmacy
http://dchealth.dc.gov/prof_license/

Florida Board of Pharmacy
http://www.doh.state.fl.us/mqa/pharmacy/pshome.htm

Georgia State Board of Pharmacy
http://www.sos.state.ga.us/plb/pharmacy/

Hawaii State Board of Pharmacy
http://www.state.hi.us/dcca/pvl/areas_pharmacy.html

Idaho Board of Pharmacy
http://www.state.id.us/bop

Illinois Department of Professional Regulation
http://www.dpr.state.il.us

Indiana Board of Pharmacy
http://www.in.gov/hpb/boards/isbp

Iowa Board of Pharmacy Examiners
http://www.state.ia.us/ibpe

Kansas State Board of Pharmacy
http://www.ink.org/public/pharmacy

Kentucky Board of Pharmacy
http://www.pharmacy.ky.gov

Louisiana Board of Pharmacy
http://www.labp.com

Maine Board of Pharmacy
http://www.state.me.us/pfr/led/ledhome2.htm
http://www.state.me.us/pfr/olr

Maryland Board of Pharmacy
http://www.dhmh.state.md.us/pharmacyboard/
related/states.htm

Massachusetts Board of Registration in
Pharmacy
http://www.state.ma.us/reg/boards/ph

Michigan Board of Pharmacy
http://www.michigan.gov/cis

Minnesota Board of Pharmacy
http://www.phcybrd.state.mn.us

Mississippi State Board of Pharmacy
http://www.mbp.state.ms.us

Missouri Board of Pharmacy
http://www.ecodev.state.mo.us/pr/pharmacy

Montana Board of Pharmacy
http://www.discoveringmontana.com

Nebraska Board of Examiners in Pharmacy
http://www.hhs.state.ne.us

Nevada State Board of Pharmacy
http://www/state.nv.us/pharmacy

New Hampshire Board of Pharmacy
http://www.state.nh.us/pharmacy

New Jersey State Board of Pharmacy
http://www.state.nj.us/lps/ca/brief/pharm.htm

New Mexico Board of Pharmacy
http://www.state.nm.us/pharmacy

New York Board of Pharmacy
http://www.nysed.gov/prof/pharm.htm

North Carolina Board of Pharmacy
http://www.ncbop.org

North Dakota State Board of Pharmacy
http://www.nodakpharmacy.com/

Ohio State Board of Pharmacy
http://www.state.oh.us/pharmacy

Oklahoma State Board of Pharmacy
http://www.state.ok.us/~pharmacy

Oregon State Board of Pharmacy
http://www.pharmacy.state.or.us

Pennsylvania State Board of Pharmacy
http://www.dos.state.pa.us/bpoa/cwp

Puerto Rico Board of Pharmacy*

Rhode Island Board of Pharmacy*

South Carolina Board of Pharmacy
http://www.llr.state.sc.us/POL/Pharmacy/

South Dakota State Board of Pharmacy
http://www.state.sd.us/dcr/pharmacy

Tennessee Board of Pharmacy
http://www..state.tn.us/commerce/boards/
pharmacy

Texas State Board of Pharmacy
http://www.tsbp.state.tx.us

Utah Board of Pharmacy
http://www.commerce.state.utah.us/dopl

Vermont Board of Pharmacy
http://www.vtprofessionals.org/pharmacists

Virgin Islands Board of Pharmacy*

Virginia Board of Pharmacy
http://dhp.state.va.us

Washington State Board of Pharmacy
http://doh.wa.gov/pharmacy

West Virginia Board of Pharmacy
http://www.wvbop.com

Wisconsin Pharmacy Examining Board
http://www.drl.state.wi.us/

Wyoming State Board of Pharmacy
http://pharmacyboard.state.wy.us

---

*No Web address

Program Costs

When determining the cost of setting up and operating a pharmacy technician program, many factors must be considered. Program designers must determine start-up costs, which include costs associated with the purchase of nonconsumable and consumable supplies, staff recruitment, program advertising, equipment, and computer hardware and software. Program maintenance costs include costs to replace consumable supplies, salaries, computer hardware and software upgrades, and student recruitment costs.

- Salary costs should be calculated for the following:
- Faculty (full-time, part-time)
- Classified staff
- Administrative staff

Costs for the following items should be included as equipment costs:

- Data projector (LCD projector for slide presentations)
- Overhead projector
- Vertical flow hood
- Laminar flow hood
- Torsion balances
- Electronic balances
- Mortar and pestles
- Counting trays and spatulas
- Prescription vials and caps (various sizes)
- Prescription bottles and caps (various sizes)
- Computers
- Small refrigerator
- Pharmacy-based software for prescription processing
- Reference books: State law book, *Facts & Comparisons*, APHA-Lexicomp Drug Information Handbook, *PDR,* and so on
- Internet access
- Consumable supplies:
    Outpatient consumables (capsules, tablets, prescription labels)
    Nonsterile compounding supplies (syrups, lactose, unibase, suppository molds, ointment jars, and so on)
    Sterile products consumables (IV bags: 250 ml, 500 ml, 1 L; medication ampules, multi-dose vials [for students to practice adding drug dose and aseptic technique])
    Miscellaneous consumables (alcohol wipes, cotton balls, and so on)

Sources of Supplies

Many program directors have been successful in procuring donations for equipment and supplies. This can significantly reduce start-up costs. Sources for donations include hospitals, home health companies, chain pharmacies, and drug distribution centers. Many of these businesses welcome the opportunity to provide resources to your program and to promote their products and services. Laminar flow hoods, vertical flow hoods, TPN compounders, computers, pharmacy-based software, vials, IV solutions, empty medicine stock vials, and torsion balances are some of the items program directors have been able to obtain as donations to their programs. Outdated medicines for counting and identification should be sought only after review of state regulations. Laws regulating possession of legend drugs without a prescription must be considered. Strict control of legend drugs is required to prevent liability associated with accidental consumption or diversion. Capsules produced by students in the nonsterile compounding course could be used for counting practice in the community practice course.

Program supplies that have not been donated or produced by students must be purchased. A list of suppliers of pharmacy equipment and supplies is provided below. The list includes suppliers of consumable and nonconsumable supplies.

Suppliers

Practice ampules (Practi-Amp)
Wallcur Inc. (800-565-4331)
San Diego, CA

Pharmacy supplies
Health Care Logistics, Inc., 800-848-1633
http://www.hcl-intl.com

Chemical, safety, laboratory products
Spectrum Laboratory Products 800-772-8786
14422 South San Pedro Street
Gardenia, CA 90248
or
755 Jersey Ave
New Brunswick, NJ 08901
http://www.spectrumchemical.com

Vertical flow hoods/laminar flow hoods, Laboratory equipment and glassware
Cole Parmer Instrument Company
www.coleparmer.com
800-323-4340
625 East Bunker Court
Vernon Hills, IL 60061-1844

Mortars, pestle, compounding supplies and equipment, patient advisory labels, vials and ointment jars, and so on
Apothecary Products, Inc
11750 12th Ave South
Burnsville, MN 55337
800-328-1584
www.apothecaryproducts.com

Software

IV labeling program by Medi-Dose called IV Profile/Label Software, $450.00, requires a dot matrix printer
Bob Braverman
rbraverman@medidose.com
www.medi-dose.com

RX30 institutional care software
Jerry Grannis
jlgrannis@earthlink.net

TechRX T-Rex One outpatient processing software, approximately $5000.00
info@techrx.com
877-800-5299

Videos

Insight Media
2162 Broadway
New York, NY 10024-0621
800-233-9910

Pharmacy Technician
Illustrates the responsibilities of pharmacy technicians in hospital, community pharmacies, and
mail order—18 min, $139

Drug Substitution: Brand Name vs Generic
Highlights differences and similarities between brand name and generic and discusses regulations
governing pharmaceutical industry—25 min, $259

Drugs
What is a drug? Overview of basic pharmacology—20 min, $109

Medication Classifications 1
Primary applications and side effects of narcotics, hypnotics, antibiotics, anticoagulants, antide-
pressants, antiarthritics, and antidiarrheals—$259

Medication Classifications 2
Primary applications and side effects of antihistamines, antineoplastics, tranquilizers, survey of
vitamins—$259

Pyxis training video, $199.00
Midwest sales person, Jeff Brannon 800-788-6245 x7320
Or Leslie Franson at Pyxis.Leslie.franson@pyxis.com

Pharmacy Technician, available through Films for the Humanities and Sciences
800-257-5126 #GDA29322, video for $89.95

Role of Pharmacy Technician: ORV
National Association Chain Drug Stores
http://www.nacds.org/

Retention

Designing a pharmacy technician program requires knowledge, dedication, and commitment to quality educational design; however, an equal challenge comes from enrollment and retention of students. Essential to program design is creation of an environment that supports student success. Many colleges and universities have institutional enrollment requirements. Failure to meet these enrollment requirements can result in course or program cancellation. Furthermore, most pharmacy technician programs receive federal, state, or local government funding. This funding is tied to training, enrollment, and retention requirements. The Workforce Investment Act of 2000 links funding levels to:

- Completion rates
- Job attainment
- Program retention
- Employment retention
- Wage satisfaction
- Nontraditional program participation

The typical student receiving educational funding through a government or company worker retraining act is a nontraditional student. Nontraditional students are older, attend school part time, work full time, and are financially independent. They may have dependents, be single parents, be a member of a minority group, be women, or have a low socioeconomic status. Nontraditional students head the list of students least likely to complete their education. The following is a list of reasons why students fail to persist:

- Nontraditional student/campus climate uncomfortable
    "My son chose Morehouse because he wanted to be in an environment where African-American men were especially valued."–Ruth Simmons, Essence Magazine *1997 Interview with Jonnetta Cole and Ruth Simmons*
- Lack of goals
- Lack of social integration

Factors That Influence Student Persistence

- Inherent intent to persist
- Attitude of student
- Institutional values and campus climate
    The initial experience at the institution, especially before and during the first quarter (session), may determine whether a student chooses to remain
- Institutional fit
    Students who feel connected to institution are more likely to remain
    "It makes me feel good that, cause I've heard that a community college isn't serious like a university. And like, wow, this community college is like hey, I'm glad I'm here. Cause I can't relate to the (negative) things they've been telling me." –NSCC student
- External factors

- Family approval of institutional choice
    Educate student's family about the need to be supportive of student, especially first-generation students (no family members have ever attended college)
- Peers
    May influence student's decision to remain
    Provide academic and emotional support

Strategies for Improving Student Persistence

1. Good student advising
    - Help students articulate clear goals
    - Advise students about courses to take and the proper sequence to take them to achieve their goals
        "The strongest impression I have right now is about the catalog. I feel like the school doesn't care. I'm coming here and I have to plan everything out and hope that I'm taking the right courses and hope that this is taking me somewhere." -frustrated NSCC student
2. Foster student involvement on and off campus
3. Link various departments, academic staff, and student services into collaborative communities in the service of student learning
4. Help students learn that they can do college-level work, that their ideas have value, and that they are worthy of respect
5. Have faculty devote time to discussing the outside concerns versus being a student. Provide information to students, especially those at risk of leaving in first quarter, of ways other students have successfully managed home, work, and school to achieve their objectives

Additional Coursework for College Success

- Goal setting
- Time management
- Note taking
- Test taking
- Critical reading

Where to Find Instructors

Before beginning the search for qualified pharmacy technician educators, it is important to ascertain the requirements of the credentialing body. For example, a board of pharmacy may require instructors be licensed pharmacists. Other credentialing bodies permit pharmacy technicians to train pharmacy technician students; however, they may want a pharmacist to be on the program advisory board. Nationally, there are programs administered and taught by pharmacists, pharmacy technicians, nurses, and professionals with degrees in education.

Instructors can be found in a variety of places. If the program director is a pharmacist or pharmacy technician, it is logical to begin the search with people he or she has worked with and whose skills and ability to communicate with staff and patients is known by the program director. Many pharmacists are licensed preceptors and have been approved by the board of pharmacy to train pharmacist students in pharmacy practice settings. If the program director is not a pharmacist or pharmacy technician, the search for qualified instructors might begin at local professional pharmacy organization such as the state chapter of the American Society of Health Systems Pharmacist (ASHP) or American Pharmaceutical Association (APhA).

Many states still permit on-the-job training of pharmacy technicians. Program directors could contact pharmacy practice settings that train pharmacy technicians to see if the on-site trainer has interest in teaching part time in the formal education program. This strategy encourages collaboration between the educational institution and employers and can ensure placement of students in externship training sites.

Future Career Opportunities and Trends

The shortage of pharmacy personnel will not end in the near future. One of the solutions to this crisis is the increased use of well-educated pharmacy support personnel. NACDS presented an interesting solution to the pharmacy's staffing crisis at the NABP Task Force on Standardization of Technician's Roles and Competencies on December 16, 1999. NACDS floated the concept of career laddering:

- Entry level technician
- Certified technician
- (A level of pharmacy technician who has training beyond most state requirements, perhaps a 2-year degree. The pharmacy technician who has achieved this level of education could also have enhanced responsibilities.)
- Pharmacist

Career laddering enables pharmacy technicians to gradually increase their education, and move from pharmacy technician to pharmacist if desired. PTEC supports career laddering and would like to see greater collaboration between schools of pharmacy and pharmacy technician programs to facilitate this career objective.

Expanded technician roles commensurate with training:

- Assist RPh with data collection
- In-house training of newly hired pharmacy technicians and pharmacy technician students
- Quality Assurance (Q&A)
- Assist in Drug Utilization Review (DUR)
- Serve on pharmacy committees
- Management of automation technology
- Inventory control
- Management of pharmacy billing
- Taking oral prescriptions
- Transferring copies of prescriptions
- Calling for refills
- Patient education (blood glucose monitor, BP measuring devices, ostomy care supplies, durable medical equipment)
- Tech-check-tech (currently 4 states permit tech-check-tech)

As previously discussed, expansion of the role of pharmacy technicians must be in concert with standardization of training and national examination to determine competency. Pharmacy technicians who have received broad-based training will be able to work in any practice setting, which is necessary if we are truly to address pharmacy technician shortages. Furthermore, comprehensive training accompanied by national certification might encourage state boards of pharmacy to consider offering reciprocity to pharmacy technicians who have been trained in other states. Reciprocity will facilitate ease of transferring to states that have pharmacy technician job shortages.

Appendix A: Essential Reading

Medication Errors Report and Recommendations, December 2000 authored by the Department of Health in response to a mandate from the Washington State Legislature. The complete report is available at: www.doh.wa.gov/mederrors/document/Reportfinal.doc

American Council on Pharmaceutical Education (ACPE) Open Hearing on Pharmacy Technician Education and Training, Annual Meeting of the American Pharmaceutical Association, New Orleans, LA March 31, 2003

Rouse, Michael, 2002 White Paper on Pharmacy Technicians
Am J Health-Syst Pharm—Vol 60 Jan 1, 2003
http://www.rxptec.org/technicianswhitepaperjan2003.pdf

Model Curriculum for Pharmacy Technician Training, ed 2, 2001 (view Model Curriculum for Pharmacy Technician Training at
http://www.ashp.org/technician/model_curriculum/index.cfm?cfid=22856876&CFToken=60041269

Ringold DJ, Santell JP, Schneider PJ. ASHP national survey of pharmacy practice in acute care settings: dispensing and administration. *Am J Health-Syst Pharm.* 2000; 57:1759-75

National Association of Chain Drug Stores, American Pharmaceutical Association, National Community Pharmacists Association. White paper. Implementing effective change in meeting the demands of community pharmacy practice in the United States, 1999

Muenzen PM, Greenberg S, Murer MM. PTCB task analysis identifies role of certified pharmacy technicians in pharmaceutical care. *J Am Pharm Assoc.* 1999; 39:857-64

Moscou K. Pharmacy technician educators' attitudes toward education and training requirements for pharmacy technicians., *J Pharm Technol.* 2000; 16:133-7

National Association of Boards of Pharmacy, Report of the Task Force on Standardization of Technicians' Roles and Competencies. 2000 May 8

Nouri L. The utilization of certified pharmacy technicians with automation and technology. Paper presented at APhA Annual Meeting. Washington, DC; 2000, Mar 12

American Society of Health-System Pharmacists Commission on Credentialing. ASHP regulations on accreditation of pharmacy technician training programs.
www.ashp.org/technicians/techregs.pdf

Appendix B: Useful Websites

National Community Pharmacists Association
http://www.ncpanet.org

National Pharmacy Technician Association
http://www.pharmacytechnican.org

Pharmacy Technician Educator Council
http://www.rxptec.org

American Pharmaceutical Association
http://aphanet.org

American Association of Pharmacy Technicians
http://www.pharmacytechnician.com

American Association of Health Systems Pharmacists
http://www.ashp.org

American Association of Colleges of Pharmacy
http://www.aacp.org

American Society of Consultant Pharmacists
http://www.ascp.com

American College of Clinical Pharmacy
http://accp.com

Academy of Managed Care Pharmacy
http://www.amcp.org/

Board of Pharmaceutical Specialties
http://www.bpsweb.org

Commission for Certification in Geriatric Pharmacy
http://www.ccgp.org

Pharmacy Education Resources, Inc.
http://www.pharmacyeducation.cc/

American College of Apothecaries
http://www.helix.com/helix/assoc/assn_pharm/aca/assn_aca.htm

Campus Compact
http://www.compact.org/

RX Trek
http://www.rxtrek.net/

Tech Lectures for Pharmacy Technicians
http://www.techlectures.com/

PharmacyTechEd
http://www.homestead.com/pharmacyteched/index.html

Powerpak CE
http://www.powerpak.com/

Professional Compounding Centers of America
http://www.pccarx.com/

RX School
http://www.rxschool.com/

Pharmcatalyst Retail Pharmacy Info
http://www.pharmcatalyst.com/

Appendix C: Professional Membership Organizations

Pharmacy Technician Educator Council
http://www.rxptec.org

American Association of Colleges of Pharmacy
http://www.aacp.org

American Association of Pharmacy Technicians
http://www.pharmacytechnician.com

American Pharmacists Association
http://www.aphanet.org

American Society of Health-System Pharmacists
http://www/ashp.org

APhA–Pharmacist.com
http://www.pharmacist.com

Canadian Association of Pharmacy Technicians
http://www.capt.ca

Joint Commission on Accreditation of Healthcare Organizations
http://www.jcaho.org

National Pharmacy Technician Association
http://www.pharmacytechnician.org

Appendix D: State Pharmacy Organizations

Alabama Pharmacy Association
http://www.aparx.org

Alabama Society of Health System
Pharmacists
http://www.alshp.org

Alaska Pharmaceutical Association
http://www.alaskapharmacy.org

Arizona Pharmacy Association
http://www.azpharmacy.org

Arizona Society of Health System
Pharmacists
http://www.azshp.org

Arkansas Association of Health System
Pharmacists
http://www.aahponline.org

California Pharmacists Association
http://www.cpha.com

California Society of Health System
Pharmacists
http://www.cshp.org

Colorado Pharmacists Association and
Colorado Society of Health System
Pharmacists
http://www.copharm.org/

Connecticut Pharmacists Association
http://www.ctpharmacists.org

Connecticut Society of Health System
Pharmacists*

Delaware Pharmacists Society Association
http://www.depharmacy.net/associations.htm

Florida Pharmacy Association
http://www.pharmview.com

Florida Society of Health System Pharmacists
http://www.fshp.org

Georgia Pharmacy Association
http://www.gpha.org

Georgia Society of Health System
Pharmacists
http://www.gshp.org

Hawaii Pharmacists Association*

Idaho Society of Health System Pharmacists
http://www.ishp.us

Idaho State Pharmacy Association
http://www.idahopharmacy.org

Illinois Council of Health-System Pharmacists
http://www.ichpnet.org

Illinois Pharmacists Association
http://www.ipha.org

Indiana Pharmacists Alliance
http://www.indianapharmacists.org

---

*No Web address

Iowa Pharmacy Association
http://www.iarx.org

Kansas Pharmacy Foundation
http://www.kansaspharmacy.org

Kansas Society of Health System Pharmacists
http://www.kansaspharmacy.org/kshp/

Kentucky Pharmacists Association
http://www.kphanet.org

Kentucky Society of Health System
    Pharmacists
http://www.kshp.org

Louisiana Pharmacists Association
http://www.louisanapharmacists.org/aboutlpa/
    index.html

Louisiana Society of Health System
    Pharmacists
http://www.lshp.org

Maine Society of Health System Pharmacists
http://www.meshp.org

Maryland Pharmacists Association
http://www.erols.com/mpha

Maryland Society of Health System
    Pharmacists
http://www.mshp.org

Massachusetts Pharmacists Association
http://www.masspharmacists.org

Massachusetts Society of Health System
    Pharmacists
http://www.mashp.org

Michigan Pharmacists Association
http://www.mipharm.com

Minnesota Pharmacists Association
http://www.mpha.org

Mississippi Pharmacists Association
http://www.mspharm.org/

Mississippi Society of Health System
    Pharmacists
http://www.pharmd.org/mshp

Missouri Pharmacy Association
http://www.morx.com

Missouri Society of Health System
    Pharmacists
http://www.moshp.com

Montana Society of Health System
    Pharmacists/Montana State
    Pharmaceutical Association
http://www.rxmt.org

Nebraska Pharmacists Association
http://www.npharm.org

Nevada Pharmacy Alliance
http://www.nvphall.org

New Hampshire Pharmacists Association
http://www.state.nh.us/pharmacy/nhpa.htm

New Jersey Pharmacists Association
http://www.njpharma.org

New Jersey Society of Health System
    Pharmacists
http://www.njshp.org/

New Mexico Pharmaceutical Association
http://www.nm-pharmacy.com

New Mexico Society of Health System
    Pharmacists
http://www.nmshp.org

New York State Council of Health System
    Pharmacists
http://www.nyschp.org

North Carolina Association of Pharmacists
http://www.ncpharmacists.org

North Dakota Pharmaceutical
    Association
http://www.ndpha@nodakpharmacy.com

North Dakota Society of Health System
    Pharmacists
http://www.nodakpharmacy.com/organizations/
    ndshp.html

Ohio Pharmacists Foundation
http://www.ohiopharmacists.org

Ohio Society of Health System Pharmacists
http://www.ohioshp.org

Oklahoma Pharmacists Association
http://www.opha.com

Oklahoma Society of Health System
  Pharmacists
http://www.oshp.net

Oregon Society of Health System
  Pharmacists
http://www.oshp.org

Pennsylvania Pharmacists Association
http://www.papharmacists.com

Pennsylvania Society of Health System
  Pharmacists
http://www.pshp.org

Pharmacy Society of Wisconsin
http://www.pswi.org

Rhode Island Society of Health System
  Pharmacists
http://www.rishp.org

South Carolina Pharmacy Association
http://www.scrx.org/scrx/

South Carolina Society of Health System
  Pharmacists
http://www.scshp.com

South Dakota Pharmacists Association
http://www.sdpha.org

Tennessee Society of Health System
  Pharmacists
http://www.tnpharm.org

Texas Pharmacy Association
http://www.txpharmacy.com

Texas Society of Health System Pharmacists
http://www.tshp.org

Utah Pharmaceutical Association
http://www.upha.com

Utah Society of Health System Pharmacists
http://www.ushp.org

Vermont Pharmacy Association
http://www.vtpharmacists.org

Virginia Pharmacists Association
http://www.vapharmacy.org/vpha

Washington State Pharmacy Association
http://www.pharmcare.org

West Virginia Pharmacists Association*

West Virginia Society of Health System
  Pharmacists
http://www.wvshp.org

Wyoming Society of Health System
  Pharmacists*

---

*No Web address